DEDICATION

I dedicate this book to eldest daughter, Andrea. She inspires me to continue writing new recipes on natural beauty.

TABLE OF CONTENTS

Natural Beauty Recipes for the Modern Woman

A Perfect Guide on How to Get that Natural Beauty

By: Susan Johnson

9781634289962

PUBLISHERS NOTES

Disclaimer – Speedy Publishing LLC

This publication is intended to provide helpful and informative material. It is not intended to diagnose, treat, cure, or prevent any health problem or condition, nor is intended to replace the advice of a physician. No action should be taken solely on the contents of this book. Always consult your physician or qualified health-care professional on any matters regarding your health and before adopting any suggestions in this book or drawing inferences from it.

The author and publisher specifically disclaim all responsibility for any liability, loss or risk, personal or otherwise, which is incurred as a consequence, directly or indirectly, from the use or application of any contents of this book.

Any and all product names referenced within this book are the trademarks of their respective owners. None of these owners have sponsored, authorized, endorsed, or approved this book.

Always read all information provided by the manufacturers' product labels before using their products. The author and publisher are not responsible for claims made by manufacturers.

This book was originally printed before 2014. This is an adapted reprint by Speedy Publishing LLC with newly updated content designed to help readers with much more accurate and timely information and data.

Speedy Publishing LLC

40 E Main Street, Newark, Delaware, 19711

Contact Us: 1-888-248-4521

Website: http://www.speedypublishing.co

REPRINTED Paperback Edition: ISBN: 9781634289962

Manufactured in the United States of America

How do you know which natural skin care products are actually safe? Some products are labeled as "100% natural" when they still contain chemicals and toxins. The only way to be completely sure is to look at the list of ingredients on the package. Dyes, fragrances, and synthetic preservatives can all be found in these "natural" skin care products.

Benefits of Natural Beauty Secrets

Women everywhere around the world are literally dying to know natural beauty secrets. As women go under the knife for one plastic surgery after another, they risk their lives and their bodies in an attempt to appear naturally beautiful. Little thought is given to how a botched surgery can affect them or their loved ones down the road. All they can think of is this unrealistic image of what's considered beautiful that they have in the heads thanks to the media and advertising.

The truth is, natural beauty secrets are not really all that secret. Everywhere a woman looks, she can find all natural ways to become someone that is truly beautiful instead of trying to imitate a digitally airbrushed and otherwise changed photograph from an ad in a magazine. A couple of the biggest secrets entail nothing more than loving yourself for precisely who you are, perceived imperfections and all.

There are so many benefits of natural beauty secrets. If you make the decision to love yourself for exactly who you are and make an effort to do so daily, your self confidence will soar. If you are happy with whom you are, you will be a happier person.

If you're a happier person, your interactions with others will be more pleasant. If you treat others more kindly, they will also be happier. The world could literally be a better place if women decided to love themselves; instead of aspiring to be something no normal woman could ever be.

Everyone wants a better quality of life. For some women, they feel that if they just looked like that model or such-and-such celebrity, they would have everything they could possibly want and more. They feel that sort of beauty will open doors for them. In reality, while beauty might open a few doors, those doors will quickly be shut if you're ugly on the inside. A woman who is dedicated to getting what she wants and feels she deserves will go much farther n this world than one who relies on her good looks alone.

Another benefit of the natural beauty secret of being happy with who you are, at the end of the day, when all is said and done, you only have yourself. If you don't like yourself as a person, you can't expect anyone else to like you, either. While some may immediately be drawn to you because of your perceived beauty, they will quickly leave once they realize how poisonous your personality is. You'll wind up alone, with only a mirror for company.

Stop letting others dictate what you should wear, how you should look, or how you should act! Don't let people who don't even know you tell you what to do with your life and body! The media and advertising executives don't know who you are. They don't even know you exist. Make the choice to do what's best for you. That is the real natural beauty secret.

Chapter 1 - Natural Beauty, Natural Skin Care

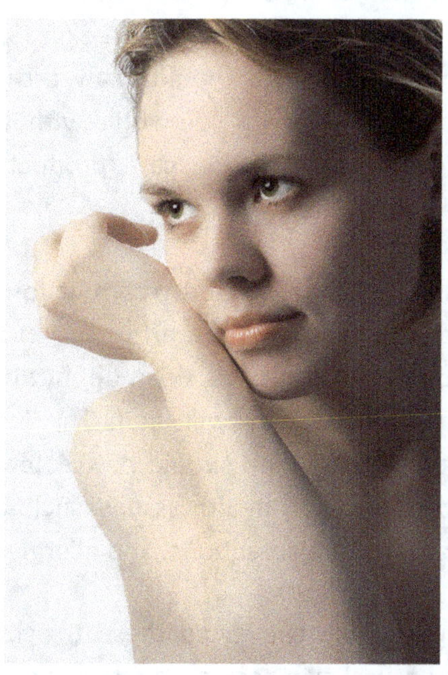

Natural skin care products may be the answer if you are concerned about the chemicals in most commercial cosmetic products. Some of these chemicals may be toxic enough to actually accelerate the aging process, which is the opposite of what you are trying to accomplish with your skin care. Even in these days of increased regulation and consumer watchdog groups, there are a number of new products introduced each year that still contain damaging chemicals.

Almost nine hundred toxic chemicals have been found in commercial cosmetic products by the National Institute of Occupational Safety and Health. The Cancer Coalition has stated that cosmetic and personal care products pose a higher threat of cancer than even smoking cigarettes. Compounding the problem is the vast amount of incorrect information distributed by marketing departments to attract new customers.

Everything that you put on the surface of your skin is absorbed into the pores and gets into the bloodstream. The circulation of the blood distributes the toxins throughout the entire body, causing damage to internal organs as well as the skin. Since all of these products enter your body, you should analyze the labels on your cosmetic products the same way you would with labels on food. Of course, choosing only natural skin care products eliminates the problem of toxins altogether.

Once the toxins get into your bloodstream, it forces your body to work much harder than usual in an effort to get rid of them. The liver is responsible for most of this clean up, but it can only handle so much before health problems will set in. The liver is a key part of the body's immune system and should be treated with care. Liver problems can cause major health issues such as auto-immune diseases, asthma, continual infections, and allergies.

Using natural ingredients can avoid these toxicity problems. The body recognizes natural skin care products as organic matter to be processed, not as a toxic threat that must be eliminated. Many of these products are made out of plant matter which contains the same basic vitamins and minerals as the ones already present in our bodies. Synthetic chemicals may be seen by the body as toxic and the immune system will react against them.

You can exfoliate with a gentle material such as crushed oatmeal, table sugar, or baking soda. Make exfoliating a regular part of your daily skin care routine and you will see much more life and bounce in your appearance. Other natural substances that may be useful for skin care include honey, egg whites, olive oil, bananas, and avocado. Be creative and use of some of the common items you have in your kitchen to give you softer, smoother skin.

CHAPTER 2- UNVEIL THE TRUTH OF NATURAL BEAUTY

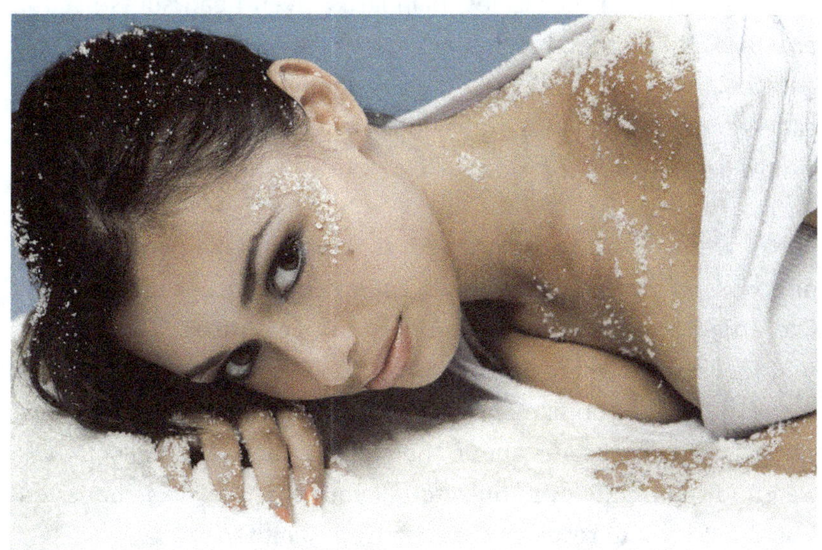

Discover the Truth about All Natural Beauty

All natural beauty is something many women want but few know they have. Instead, they get expensive surgeries done, literally risking their lives in the pursuit of a beauty standard that is not only unrealistic but is completely unreal. They use beauty products that damage their skin and hair and ultimately wind up in landfills when they don't have the promised effects. Women are hurting themselves and the environment all in an effort to be beautiful.

Fortunately, there are many different ways women can achieve the all natural beauty that they so desperately want and deserve. Some of these ways are exceptionally easy to incorporate into a womans everyday life. Some of them may be a little bit trickier for some to get used to doing everyday but once fitted into a womans daily habits, they will be easy to maintain for a lifetime.

The first step to all natural beauty is to stop idolizing the models you see in magazines or on billboards. Stop looking to female celebrities and comparing yourself to them. Nearly all advertisements in magazines, billboards, even head shots used in portfolios, have been touched up in one way or another digitally to get rid of wrinkles, acne, or other unsightly blemishes. No woman can ever live up to how a model looks in a photo because the photo simply isn't real.

Next, women everywhere need to realize how beautiful they already are. Everyone has flaws or imperfections that they don't like about themselves; even models and celebrities. You need to quit focusing on where you think you don't measure up and instead focus on things you like about yourself. For some women, finding things they appreciate about themselves can be a difficult task. Recruit friends and loved ones to tell you what they like about you. You don't have to restrict yourself to looks, either.

Which leads to the next truth about all natural beauty: it comes from within. It may sound very cliché but the phrase has existed for a long time for a reason. Beautiful personalities, feeling confident in yourself without being cocky, helping others, and honestly caring for those around you will make you a truly beautiful person. People with picture perfect bodies but who have ugly hearts and souls may lead a charmed life on the outside but on the inside; things aren't as lovely.

Because they are so mean and hurtful to those around them, they drive people away from them, and wind up alone in the end.

Surround yourself with people that are truly beautiful from the inside and you will not only be happier but you'll stop turning to a Hollywood standard that even models and celebrities can't live up to. Don't be tempted to turn into a plastic person through plastic surgery or other extreme measures in order to be a fantasy version of someone who doesn't know you exist. The truth about all natural beauty is in understanding the beauty within.

Discover the Truth About Raw Natural Beauty Products

Raw natural beauty products are known for three things: safety, performance, and prestige. The company's goal is to provide high-end skin care products that are also safe for your skin and the environment. In the past, this was thought to be impossible, as natural products were known for their low quality. This is not the case with Raw's new line of natural beauty products.

Most cosmetic companies that produce natural skin care items are only concerned with making sure the product is as natural as possible. Performance and style are often overlooked in an attempt to be authentic. Raw Natural Beauty combines performance with practicality and shows that an organic brand can also be a high-end luxury product.

Raw natural beauty products were developed after extensive market research into what women really wanted from their cosmetics. The overwhelming response was that they wanted performance and quality over all else. Price was important, as were natural ingredients, but these factors are moot if the cosmetics do not perform adequately. So, not only are Raw's natural beauty products designed to outperform the rest of the natural cosmetics market, they are also intended to compete with traditional, commercial cosmetic products.

The natural beauty niche has had a bad reputation as low-end, homemade products using items from the kitchen. Raw Natural Beauty shows that it is possible to create effective products out of natural ingredients without losing performance. This performance comes as a result of even more research, this time into new ingredients from around the world that can be used to improve the products.

Natural Beauty line contains these exotic, natural, active botanicals clinically proven to improve the skin over time. This is something I have not seen yet from any other brand, natural or not.

In seeking out these ingredients, Raw natural beauty further demonstrates its commitment to the environment and green business practices. They only use suppliers who practice sustainable agriculture to minimize the environmental damage caused by the production of their cosmetics. Vendors who are frequent donators in their community and support fair trade practices are also looked upon favorably when deciding where to purchase supplies.

Safety of ingredients is also a top priority for Raw Natural Beauty. In fact, most people would say that it's the ingredient safety that leads them to purchase a natural product over a mainstream cosmetic product. However, natural does not automatically mean an ingredient is safe, so Raw takes it a step further and tests each and every one of its ingredients against a national safety rating database.

Raw Natural Beauty has also signed off on the Compact for Safe Cosmetics, which cements their commitment to using only safe ingredients that are not known to be toxic. Whatever is put on the surface of the skin is eventually absorbed and metabolised by the body, so it is very important to use only safe skin care products. With all of their safeguarding and testing, you can be sure you are getting only the best ingredients from Raw Natural Beauty.

CHAPTER 3- NATURAL BEAUTY – HOW TO CHOOSE THE RIGHT SKIN CARE PRODUCTS

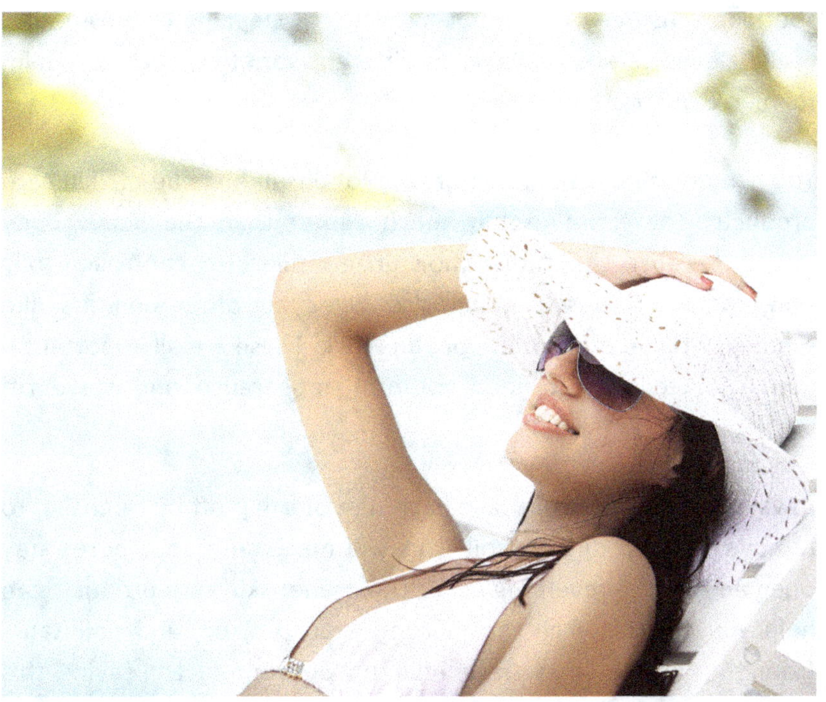

The right set of skin care products can show the world that you care about your appearance and what you use on your skin. After all, your face is the first thing people see when they meet you, so you want to look your best. Here are some things to look for when trying to protect your skin.

Simply washing your face with soap alone is not sufficient daily skin care. Soap may clean up some of the oil and dirt on your face and may even open up some pores, but it does nothing to moisturize or condition your skin. In addition to your normal daily routine of washing with soap, add in some quality skin care products to protect and soften your skin.

There are a number of facial care products on the market to choose from. Always use a facial cleanser instead of regular bar soap because body soap can dry out the face and will not give you any of the moisturizing properties of a good cleanser. Specially designed cleansers can be used for treating oily or dry skin, soothing sensitive skin, removing acne, or cleaning off cosmetics. Facial cleansers are available in different varieties, such as liquid, foam, cream, or gel.

You can also find a selection of face lotions in any line of skin care products. These are usually much lighter than the heavy body lotions because they must moisturize while also controlling oily skin. Many of these lotions also give you other benefits like tanning, wrinkle prevention, or sun block. These are all important if you want to protect your youthful appearance and stave off wrinkles.

Always take care of your face each day, starting off by cleansing to remove built up dirt and oil. This will make sure your pores stay open and clear, preventing acne. The proper skin care products can help you get rid of all that accumulated dirt, oil, and pollutants from the air that may have built up on your face. Leaving this untreated may lead to more serious skin problems or even infection if the buildup is too great.

Specialized skin care products are also available to deal with conditions like eczema, blackheads, and whiteheads. There are wipes, pads, gels, creams, foams, and more that are all individually designed to handle a certain skin condition. To clean out the pores overnight, you can get a facial mask that hardens on the skin and peels off with all of the impurities. Check the instructions that come with the product as some require the mask to be rinsed off and others simply can be peeled off.

For more luxurious skin care treatment, you can go to a spa for a full-service facial. In addition to facial services, most spas offer body massages and saunas so you can also unwind and reduce stress. While these high-end services may be expensive, you can usually get a basic facial for a reasonable price at most spas. Also, a quality spa should have the latest in skin care products for you to purchase for your own home use.

Natural Beauty Tips to Help You Look Your Best

Let our natural beauty tips help you look beautiful without all those toxic chemicals found in today's cosmetics. It is possible to achieve a healthy, vibrant appearance using only natural ingredients. You'll look better and feel better because you do not have all those heavy cosmetic products on your skin.

Natural beauty refers to a vital and healthy look for your body, hair, and skin. Living an overall healthier lifestyle is the first step to refreshing your appearance. Take care of your body from the inside out before attempting to fix skin problems with surface treatments like moisturizer or makeup. Many times, a simple lifestyle change is all it takes to completely revitalize your look.

Make sure you are eating right and are getting enough vitamins and minerals each day. Add a multivitamin to your morning routine to ensure that you are receiving all the nutrients your body needs. Eat plenty of fruits and vegetables and try to avoid excess fats, sugars, and processed foods. Healthy food for your body will show through in your appearance as your skin clears and becomes more moist and supple.

Exercise is probably the most powerful of any of the natural beauty tips. Regular physical activity improves blood flow to the skin, giving it a fuller, more colorful look naturally. Of course, exercise will also help you stay trim and looking good all-around. On top of the benefits to your appearance, working out on a regular basis will keep your internal organs and heart healthy, along with preventing some cancers and extending your life.

The next in our list of natural beauty tips is to always keep yourself hydrated. As skin dries out, it becomes inflexible and more susceptible to wrinkles. Instead of applying heavy moisturizing cream externally, try drinking more water to provide moisture from the inside. This is a far healthier and natural solution to the common problem of dry skin.

Even if you still want to wear some cosmetics, there are natural beauty tips that can help you. Start off with either a sheer foundation or a slightly tinted moisturizing cream. Use a damp sponge to apply the cream so you get coverage all over your face without too much cosmetic buildup. This shows off your healthy-looking skin, but will also cover up any blemishes or marks without being too heavy or obvious.

To avoid leathery, dry skin, stay out of the sun whenever possible. The UV rays from the sun will dry out your skin and cause it to wrinkle prematurely. If you must go out in direct sunlight, be sure to wear sunscreen that is rated SPF 15 or higher. Hats, sunglasses, and umbrellas can also help protect you when you are out in the sun.

As you can see it does not require chemical-filled cosmetics and makeup to look great. There are many ways to enhance your appearance without resorting to artificial products. Following these natural beauty tips will get you on your way to a healthier, more radiant appearance.

The green movement and global warming have people everywhere in search of natural health and beauty recipes. As more and more people discover these all natural recipes, more and more people decide to make them at home instead of spending the money to buy similar products from the various beauty and health stores. Who can blame them? These sorts of products tend to be more expensive than their toxic counterparts. If you make them at home, you'll save money and the environment.

Part of the problem is, as most people embark down the path of making natural health and beauty recipes, they have little to no experience in making them. People can then become discouraged and give up trying to make them at home, finding it easier and cheaper to just go back to their old, planet destroying habits. Before you throw in the towel, there are several techniques that can help give a successful result on any of the recipes you try.

Actually the first thing anyone should do when deciding to make any of the natural health and beauty recipes they find is to do some research. The internet is a great resource in learning about the ingredients used in the recipes and where to find them. You can also find tips and tricks from people who have made the recipe before, allowing you to learn from their experience and mistakes before you attempt to make it yourself. Why learn the hard way and make your own mistakes when you can learn from someone else's?

Next, you'll want to purchase a good reference book on natural health and beauty recipes. It's not always possible to hop on the internet and look up the information you need when you're right in the middle of creating something. A good reference book is also great for researching any particular ailments that might spring up on you suddenly. Having one on essential oils is a must since essential oils are used quite frequently in these sorts of recipes.

Since quite a few natural health and beauty recipes are cooked much like regular, food recipes, you'll want to purchase separate cook wear that will be used when you make your beauty recipes. Some ingredients can do wonders for a complexion but cause serious problems if ingested. It can be hard to get a pot completely clean and free of any essential oil or plant residue once it's been used for a beauty recipe. You'll avoid the likelihood of cross-contamination all together if you simply use different cook wear for different things.

When you're ready to make one of the beauty recipes, gather all of your ingredients and the recipe together, much like when you cook normally. Make sure you keep your work area clean and wipe up any spills immediately. Have whatever containers ready that you plan on storing your creation in. Natural health and beauty recipes aren't hard to do. They can be a lot of fun!

The Benefits of Professional Skin Care

You can get a variety of professional skin care products just about anywhere these days. It used to be that you were limited to only the selection of products at your local spa, but now there are quality skin care products at the pharmacy or health store, along with a number of outlets online. You no longer have to pay expensive spa fees just to get the products you need.

Along with the expanded choice of retailers, there is a vast array of professional skin care products available. You can choose an entire product line to cover all of your personal care needs or just select single products as you need them. There are also more organic and natural beauty products on the market now than ever before, so you do not have to use chemical-based skin care products. Some products have blended the natural with some synthetic substances, trying to avoid using the most toxic chemicals.

Many of these products can be purchased over the counter with no prescription, but some of the stronger items may require a prescription from a dermatologist. These products are usually a stronger concentration that is meant only for certain skin problems. They must be restricted because they may cause damage to people who do not have that particular condition. Some of the more common prescription products are used to treat acne, discoloration, and premature aging.

Of course, if you do need a prescription product, you will have to make an appointment with a dermatologist. A qualified dermatologist is the best person to decide if you have a severe enough skin condition to warrant treatment with professional skin care products. If he does determine that you have a problem, the dermatologist can suggest certain products that will be best suited for that specific skin condition. The doctor can also advise you on the safe use of all cosmetic products, including warnings specific to pregnant women.

Any professional skin care product you buy should come with an instruction booklet and warnings. A good dermatologist will also verbally warn you of any side effect and should explain how to use the product correctly. Always follow the doctor's instructions or ask the pharmacist if you have any questions about how the product should be used or how much to use.

Although all professional skin care products come with their own instruction leaflets, your dermatologist should be able to verbally repeat product instructions and warnings. A good doctor will always warn you if you should expect some side effects. He can also tell you exactly how to safely get the most out of your product. You should also check with your doctor to make sure there are no adverse reactions with any other medications or products you are currently using.

The expansion of the skin care industry has brought many high-end products to the consumer. You may now be able to find your skin care solution without having to see the dermatologist. Of course, be careful when purchasing your own products without a doctor's guidance as there may be side effects or interactions. Always do your research to make sure you are getting the right type of professional skin care products.

The Professionals Guide To Sensitive Skin Care

Sensitive skin care is a challenge for many people, especially those living in difficult climates. There are certain external conditions that should be avoided, as should the chemicals in most commercial cosmetic products. How do you know if you have sensitive skin? Here are a few factors to consider when deciding if you need specialized sensitive skin care products:

* Do you break out or have redness after being exposed to environmental stressors like shaving or weather?

* Do you have tingly or tight skin with no other explanation for it?

* Have you noticed any dryness, irritation, or redness on your skin?

* Does your skin react adversely to household cleaning products or cosmetics?

* After answering the rest of these questions, has your dermatologist ruled out any other skin conditions that could be causing the problem?

Sensitive skin can be even more challenging to deal with in adverse weather conditions. If you live where the weather is extremely cold or hot, you may need to use sensitive skin care products to protect yourself.

Thin skin is generally more sensitive than thicker parts of the skin simply because there is less protection between the blood and the outside conditions. The capillaries are closer to the outside of the skin when it is thin, so the skin becomes sensitive to cold, heat, and wind. Sensitive skin also is more susceptible to sunburn, so wear a higher SPF sunscreen if you much go out in the sun.

Avoid harsh washing products like loofahs, brushes, or cleansing stones. You want something soft to take care of your sensitive skin, not an abrasive brush that will further irritate it. Do not use exfoliants because they may be too rough for your skin and cause inflammation when used.

Stay away from any strong chemicals in your skin care products. Fragrances and dyes in particular may irritate sensitive skin, so look for hypo-allergenic or organic products whenever possible. Use liquid cleansers as they are usually easier on the skin and will not cause the same allergic reactions. Hard-milled soaps also work well for sensitive skin care.

Antibacterial astringents are another key component of a good sensitive skin care program. They come in both cream and lotion form and are used to protect your skin from infectious bacteria. This balances your skin growth and keeps bacterial colonies from forming on the surface. One strong antibacterial is salicylic acid, which can exfoliate and remove the outer layer of accumulated dead skin cells. It also clears out bacteria in hair follicle areas to ensure healthy hair growth.

Be careful when purchasing your sensitive skin care products to make sure that they really are safe for your skin. Many products are labeled as natural or hypo-allergenic when they still contain toxic chemicals. Always check the ingredients listed on the label to see if there are any substances that may aggravate your skin. Similarly, perfume-free products may not always be completely devoid of fragrances so double-check all of your sensitive skin care products before use.

CHAPTER 4- NATURAL BEAUTY – USEFUL TIPS ABOUT NATURAL BEAUTY PRODUCTS

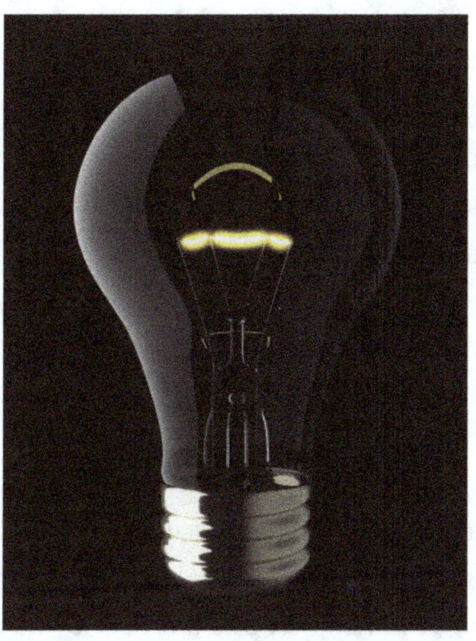

With so many dangerous chemicals in mainstream cosmetics these days, more and more women are turning to the idea of natural beauty. Natural beauty is the practice of using only organic ingredients for skin and hair care. This avoids many of the health and allergy issues caused by commercial personal care products. Here are a few tips on how to choose natural beauty products.

If you are ready to get rid of those chemical-laden cosmetic products and enter the world of natural beauty, there are quite a few choices out there. You can often save money by making your own cosmetic products at home out of common kitchen goods. When you first begin a regimen of natural products, your body may go through a brief detoxifying period while it adjust to not being drenched with toxins on a daily basis.

The face is often more sensitive than the skin on the rest of the body and must be treated accordingly. Look for a cleanser that does not dry the skin and is not too harsh. Castile soap or glycerin both work very well for cleaning the face without robbing it of precious moisture. Whatever type of cleanser you choose, be sure not to let your skin become dry and cracked, as this can lead to wrinkles.

Adding exfoliation to your daily skin care routine can help boost your skin's vibrancy and vitality. Exfoliating removes the top layer of dead skin that accumulates over time. This dead material can choke off the oxygen and sunlight to the healthy skin below and gives your face a dull appearance. Exfoliating before cleansing will strip off this unnecessary layer and let your natural beauty shine through.

Always keep your skin protected from the damaging rays of the sun. Direct sunlight can burn out the pigmentation in certain spots of the skin, leading to unsightly age spots and white patches. There are many natural sunscreens available today, many of them consisting of simple ingredients like olive oil. Of course, staying out of the sun is your best bet, but a natural beauty product with sun protection can limit the damage if you must go out.

Natural hair coloring is also available as a healthier alternative to chemical-based dyes. Throughout history, natural products have been used to spice up appearance by changing hair color. Natural hair colorings give you the option of a more mellow, subtle color change or a more drastic change, depending on the material used as a dye. Using a tea rinse gives that nice, gentle look and something like henna can give you a brighter color that really pops.

It can be confusing at first, but making the change to natural beauty products is well worth the effort. It is easy to find information these days, with the accessibility of the Internet. Local health food stores or even pharmacies may have the latest natural cosmetic products as well. With so many options, there is no reason to continue using chemical-based commercial products instead of those that bring out your natural beauty.

Learn How to Make Natural Beauty Products at Home

Want to know how to make natural beauty products at home? There are a number of natural beauty recipes you can prepare with just a few items you may already have in your kitchen. Not only are these products easy to make, but they are also healthier than using commercial products full of chemicals.

By learning how to make natural beauty products of your own, you will helping the environment, along with saving money. Most of the commercial cosmetic products on the market include some type of chemical or detergent. When this is washed off your skin or thrown in the trash, these chemicals and toxins can get into the water supply. Making your own natural beauty products out of common household items is a much greener solution.

Some common kitchen items that can be used to make natural beauty products are Epsom salt, bananas, honey, oatmeal, olive and vegetable oils, yogurt, mayonnaise. This is just a short list of household products that can be used for skin or hair care. There are quite a few other natural products that can do wonders for your appearance.

There are two common ingredients that you probably will not have on hand when you are learning how to make natural beauty products. These are beeswax and natural soap bars. Beeswax and other natural waxes can be found at health food stores, soap making shops, and some craft stores. For those allergic to bees, there are other vegetable- and flower-based waxes to choose from.

Olive oil is a very versatile home remedy that can be used for a number of natural beauty purposes. It will moisturize the dry skin of your elbows, cuticles, knees, and feet. Olive oil can be added to a warm bath for even more moisture and softness. For dry hair or scalp, simply massage the oil directly in with your hands.

You can even make your own natural exfoliating treatment from olive oil. Mix the oil with twice as much brown sugar to create a thick paste. Use this paste as a pre-shower skin treatment by rubbing gently into the skin. Rinse thoroughly in the shower to remove all paste and any dead skin cells that may have been scraped off.

If you have bananas on hand, you can also use those as a moisturizer for dry and cracked skin. Mash a ripe banana until it becomes a paste that is smooth enough to apply to your face or hands. Let the paste soak in for about ten minutes, then rinse off and pat dry. For added moisturizing, add in a teaspoon of olive oil before applying to dry, parched skin.

These are just a few of the beauty products you can make at home without spending much money. Other great home remedies include facial cleansers, herbal bath soaks, skin butter, and natural body scrubs. Most of these recipes can be made with simple ingredients that you already have at home. Now that you know how easy it is, jump right in and learn how to make natural beauty products of your own.

Natural skin care products may be the answer if you are concerned about the chemicals in most commercial cosmetic products. Some of these chemicals may be toxic enough to actually accelerate the aging process, which is the opposite of what you are trying to accomplish with your skin care. Even in these days of increased regulation and consumer watchdog groups, there are a number of new products introduced each year that still contain damaging chemicals.

Almost nine hundred toxic chemicals have been found in commercial cosmetic products by the National Institute of Occupational Safety and Health. The Cancer Coalition has stated that cosmetic and personal care products pose a higher threat of cancer than even smoking cigarettes. Compounding the problem is the vast amount of incorrect information distributed by marketing departments to attract new customers.

Everything that you put on the surface of your skin is absorbed into the pores and gets into the bloodstream. The circulation of the blood distributes the toxins throughout the entire body, causing damage to internal organs as well as the skin. Since all of these products enter your body, you should analyze the labels on your cosmetic products the same way you would with labels on food. Of course, choosing only natural skin care products eliminates the problem of toxins altogether.

Once the toxins get into your bloodstream, it forces your body to work much harder than usual in an effort to get rid of them. The liver is responsible for most of this clean up, but it can only handle so much before health problems will set in. The liver is a key part of the body's immune system and should be treated with care. Liver problems can cause major health issues such as auto-immune diseases, asthma, continual infections, and allergies.

Using natural ingredients can avoid these toxicity problems. The body recognizes natural skin care products as organic matter to be processed, not as a toxic threat that must be eliminated. Many of these products are made out of plant matter which contains the same basic vitamins and minerals as the ones already present in our bodies. Synthetic chemicals may be seen by the body as toxic and the immune system will react against them.

You can exfoliate with a gentle material such as crushed oatmeal, table sugar, or baking soda. Make exfoliating a regular part of your daily skin care routine and you will see much more life and bounce in your appearance. Other natural substances that may be useful for skin care include honey, egg whites, olive oil, bananas, and avocado. Be creative and use of some of the common items you have in your kitchen to give you softer, smoother skin.

How do you know which natural skin care products are actually safe? Some products are labeled as "100% natural" when they still contain chemicals and toxins. The only way to be completely sure is to look at the list of ingredients on the package. Dyes, fragrances, and synthetic preservatives can all be found in these "natural" skin care products.

CHAPTER 5- NATURAL BEAUTY: ONE OF THE BEST NATURAL BEAUTY RECIPES

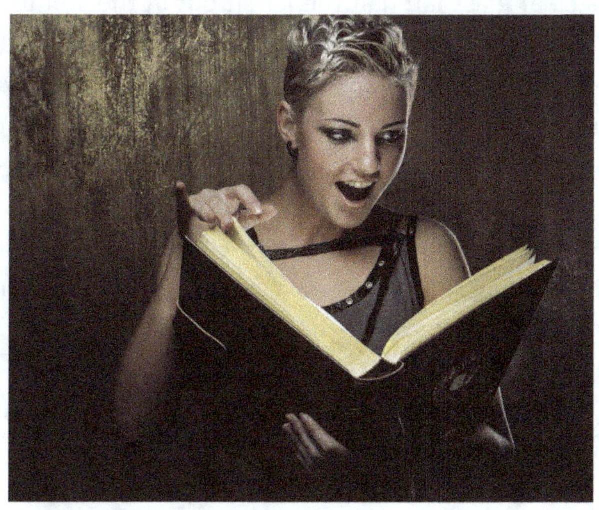

There are a number of natural beauty recipes you can make at home. You do not have to pay for commercial cosmetic products to look your best. In fact, many times the natural solution is healthier and more effective than the chemical-laden make-ups you will find at the store.

Here is a great papaya enzyme facial mask that is one of the more popular natural beauty recipes. You will need the following ingredients: 1/2 cup mashed papaya, 1 whipped egg white, and 1 teaspoon of honey. For additional cooling or if you have sensitive skin, add a tablespoon of plain yogurt to your mixture.

Mix all of your ingredients together in a large bowl. Wash your skin before applying the facial mask mixture. Leave the mask on your face for approximately five to eight minutes, giving the papaya enzymes time to exfoliate your skin. Rinse off with warm water first, then with cooler water, patting dry when done.

For hair, this herbal vinegar rinse will restore your hair's natural pH balance, clean off built up dirt and hair products, and reduce oily hair. Place 2 sprigs of rosemary and 2 sprigs of lavender in 2 cups of water in a clear glass jar. Let the jar sit out in the sun to steep for between two and four hours, then remove the herbs. Add one or two tablespoons of either apple cider vinegar or white vinegar to your water solution, then use the same way you would use shampoo.

Herbal bath salts are another of the top natural beauty recipes you can make at home. All you need is a cup of sea salt and a handful of whatever herbs you have on hand, such as lavender, rosemary, spearmint, or peppermint. Grind the herbs with a coffee grinder until they become a fine powder. Mix with the sea salt and dump into your next bath for a relaxing change of pace.

A similar natural beauty recipe is this refreshing flower-based foot soak. For this one, you again need sea salt, along with some fresh sliced citrus of your choice (limes, lemons, oranges, etc.) and a handful of flower petals picked fresh from your garden. Fill a small basin with lukewarm water and add the salt, flower petals, and fruit slices. Soak your feet in the mixture for ten minutes, then rinse and pat to dry.

This strawberry manicure mask is a great way to pamper your hands naturally. Mash 3-5 ripe strawberries, drain off the juice, and combine with one tablespoon of sugar and a little bit of the light oil of your choice. Apply the resulting mixture to your hands by using a circular motion. This will condition and exfoliate the skin, leaving it soft and smooth.

During watermelon season, this pedicure polish is good for your feet and gives your home a nice aroma of summer. Combine 1/2 cup of mashed and strained watermelon with one tablespoon finely crushed almonds and 1/4 cup of plain yogurt. Apply the mixture by working it in with your hands in a circular motion. Use a tissue to remove, then rinse and pat dry to enjoy this one of our natural beauty recipes.

What You Need to Know About Organic Skin Care

Because today's consumers are more conscious of their health and the environment, there are more organic skin care products available than ever before. Other people may have developed allergies to all of the toxins and chemicals used in commercial skin care products and are looking for a healthier alternative. Some commonly used ingredients in commercial products include fragrances, dyes, and various types of acids.

By contrast, organic skin care products contain natural ingredients such as vitamins A, C, or E, essential oils, antioxidants, or proteins. These are necessary to replace the skin cells lost as we age. As the body gets older, it produces less collagen and elastin, which leads to dry, wrinkled skin. Re-hydrating the cells from the outside is the only way to repair this age-related damage.

You can now find organic skin care products in almost any pharmacy, drug store, or health food and nutrition store. If you do not have access to any of these places, there are many retailers online to choose your natural cosmetics from. Some spas and salons have also added organic products to their inventory, so you may want to look there as well. Most of these products are free of fragrances and dyes and will not cause or aggravate existing allergies.

There are organic products available both men and women. Men can find organic shaving lotion and after-shave, while women usually have more options of cleansers, creams, toners, and gels.

Unfortunately, organic products generally cost more than the synthetic version of the same item. It is worth the extra cost to protect your skin and your health from toxic chemicals and preservatives.

An alarming number of mainstream skin care products may contain the wetting agents diethanolamine and triethanolamine, sometimes listed on ingredient labels as DEA and TEA, respectively. These substances by themselves are not considered to be a cancer risk. If the product contains nitrites as contaminants, this may cause a chemical reaction that creates cancer-causing nitrosamines.

Most commercial cosmetic products include some type of bactericides or preservatives. These are necessary to protect the cosmetics from contamination, but may also be dangerous or even carcinogenic. For instance, trace amounts of formaldehyde are found in some products. Formaldehyde is a known carcinogen and is neurotoxin in higher doses.

How can you be sure that your skin care products are really organic? Unfortunately, there is still plenty of room for vagueness in labeling of cosmetic products. Generally, a cosmetic product must follow the same USDA rules as would a food product. The product must contain no less than 95% organic and natural ingredients in order to qualify for the label.

After the 95% threshold is met, there is a serious lack of additional guidance and regulations. There are no restrictions on the words cosmetic manufacturers can use on their labels, so you many see plenty of products called "organic" or "botanical" even though they may still contain a small amount of synthetic chemicals. Read the ingredient labels carefully to be sure that your organic skin care products are really made of only organic materials.

CHAPTER 6- NATURAL BEAUTY: BASIC TIPS IN CARING FOR YOUR HAIR

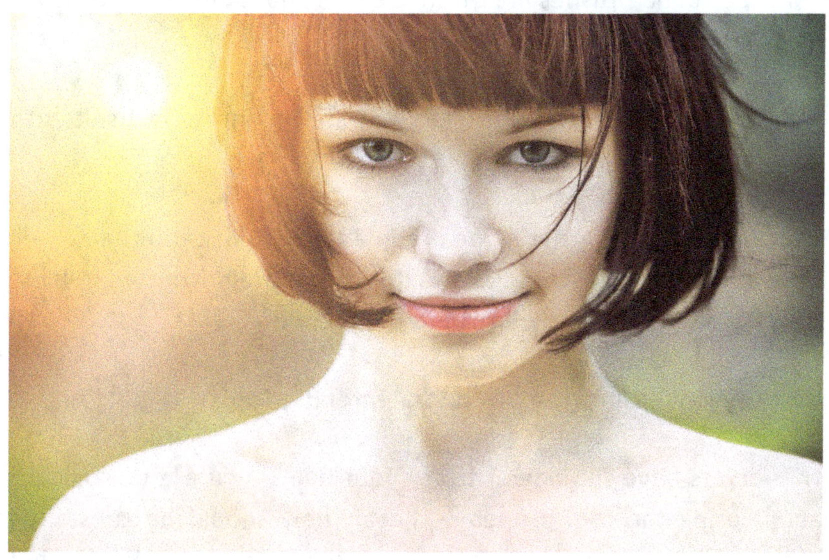

The Right Tools for the Trade

There is a tool for every job that can make life easier for you, whether it is a microwave to heat up food or the telephone to keep you in touch with the rest of the world. In the world of hair care however, there are so many products that sometimes, it is a hit or miss as to whether or not you have the right tools for your beauty regiment. And since each person and their hair is different, what works for you will not work for someone else. So if you are a little lost in this world of hair care, listed below are some of the basics that can get you through:

Brushes and Combs With a head of wet hair, you should never, ever use a brush of any kind, especially if you have tangles. The brushes will grab at your hair, tearing or breaking it, causing split ends and other damage. Only a wide toothed comb will suffice. Your hair brush is an important part of your beauty routine. There are a variety of different brushes that achieve different hair styles, depending on their use.

•Bristled round brushes are often used for those with curly or wavy hair that they wish to blow dry straight.

•A paddle brush is great for every day styling and is best suited to people with long hair.

•A vented brush is great if you are in a hurry to dry your hair. They have a vented head that allows the heated air from your blow dryer to pass through the brush to dry the hair.

Hair Dryers, Curling Irons, and Straightening Tools

Hair dryers have the power to fry your hair if you are not diligent about using the tool properly. The air flow should be constantly moving, rather than centering on one location. When that happens, damaged hair is the result. Hair dryers have attachments like diffusers that will distribute the heat in a wider area to avoid damage. There are also hair dryers that use negative ion technology to cut the drying time in half and with less damage.

Curling irons and straightening tools also have the power to damage your hair. Choose these tools wisely by selecting ones that have various levels of temperature control as well as automatic shutoff mechanisms in case you forget to unplug them. For an optimal performing curling iron or straightening tool, go with those that are made with ceramic technology. Ceramic is less likely to burn your hair and it will even provide some conditioning as it heats your hair into shape.

Shampoos

Your scalp should dictate what type of shampoo you use. If you have dandruff, you would need something specific to that condition. Oily or dry hair also dictates what type of shampoo to use. You need to shampoo every time you wash your hair to get rid of the dirt and other pollutants that you might pick up in the course of your day. Be careful and try to avoid any shampoos that have any type of alcohol in the ingredients. Alcohol can dry out your hair.

Conditioners

There is some debate as to whether or not you even need conditioner. For the most part, you do, unless you have super fine hair that looks lifeless when you use a conditioner. Hair care products, brushing, drying, curling and straightening your hair can be damaging, not to mention colors or perms. A conditioner can replenish and protect your hair from these damaging elements. To avoid oily or dull looking hair on the crown of your head, only apply conditioner to the length of your hair and avoid the scalp.

Hairsprays and Other Styling Products

A few decades ago, hairsprays had the power to eat through a hole in the ozone layer. These days, they are more environmentally friendly without harsh chemicals. The hairspray of today can protect against humid conditions and even the sun's harmful UV rays. There are a variety of formulas depending on what styles you hope to achieve.

Mousses, gel and shine serums are great for those people who have problems achieve a smooth finish without compromising any bounce and body in their hair. If you have fine hair, mousses are light and work best for the hair. With thicker heads of hair, gels work the best. Shine serums are for those people who have dull looking hair, even when it is clean. Shine serums can also sometimes perform double-duty as a frizz controller.

When in doubt, talk with your stylist about what products would best suit your hair. Ask questions each time they use a different product in your hair to achieve a certain look. They can guide you through that confusing maze of hair care tools.

Dry and Damaged Hair

The average human head has 150,000 hairs, and, conformists that they are, when one's dry, they're all dry. But unlike a dry flower garden or polished rice, the solution is not simply to add water. Water, in fact, may be responsible for the hair's parched condition, particularly if we're talking about water of the salty, chlorinated, or sudsy variety. The market is flooded with products for dry, overheated, and damaged hair, from shampoos, conditioners, to protectant masks. It can be a daunting task to know which product is right for you. Home remedies might be your best bet for having a more manageable mane.

Swimming and over-shampooing are two common causes of arid, fly-away locks. Other culprits can include colorings, permanents, electric curlers, excessive blow-drying, and too much exposure to wind and sun. Keep your styling products and accessories to a minimum to keep from drying out your locks completely.

Whatever the culprit, your poor, abused hair needs help—badly. You can almost hear all 150,000 of them down on their little split ends, pleading, "Save me! Save me!" Here's a quick course on how to rescue dried-out hair.

Shampoo with Care

"It's in vogue these days to shampoo every day, but shampooing doesn't only wash away dirt, it washes out the hair's protective oils," says Thomas Goodman, Jr., M.D. If you've dried your hair out from too much lather, give your hair a needed break—try washing less often. And use only a mild shampoo, one labeled "for dry or damaged hair."

Use a Conditioner

When hair becomes dry, the outer layers, called cuticles, peel off from the central shaft. Conditioners glue the cuticles back to the shaft, add lubricant to the hair, and prevent static electricity (which creates frizz). Pick a conditioner that works well for you and use it after every shampoo, says Dr. Goodman.

Go Heavy on the Mayo

Mayonnaise makes an excellent conditioner. Leave the oily white goo in your hair for anywhere from 5 minutes to an hour before washing it out.

Snip Off Those Frayed Ends

Dry hair tends to suffer most at the ends. What is the answer? Snip 'em off. Get a trim every six weeks or so to keep those frayed ends under control.

Design Your Hair Without Heat

Heat is what makes the desert a desert; it also contributes to dried-out hair. Two of the most intense sources of heat are curling irons and electric curlers. It is suggested by top Hollywood hairstylists that you rediscover those (unheated) plastic cylinder rollers from years gone by. For straightening, wrap slightly moist hair under and around rollers (like a page boy hairdo) for about 10 minutes. For curling or adding wave, try using sponge rollers overnight or sleeping with moist braids.

Protect Your Hair from the Elements

Whipping wind can fray your hair just like a piece of fabric. Sun, too, takes a mighty toll. Solution: Wear a hat, both on breezy, balmy summer days, and gusty, frosty winter days.

Don't Swim Bare Headed

Chlorine is one of the most destructive things to hair. So make a rubber cap part of your regular swim attire. For extra protection first rub a little olive oil into your hair.

Have a Beer

Beer is a wonderful setting lotion. It gives a crisp, healthy, shiny look, even to dry hair. The trick is to spray the brew onto your hair using a pump bottle after you've shampooed and towel-dried, but before you blow-dry or style. And don't worry about smelling like a lush—the odor of the beer quickly disappears.

Consider a Trip to the Beauty Parlor

Experts agree that a professional moisturizing treatment can work wonders for your dried-out head of hair. A real good steam treatment with oils and creams lasts about an hour, and afterward you can really tell the difference. If you can't afford a salon beauty treatment, get a store-bought intensive conditioning treatment to bring some moisture back into your locks.

Drink Plenty of Water and Eat Raw Fruits

What you put into your body is reflected on the outside especially in your hair.

Mash up some rotten bananas and avocados

This makes a nutrient-rich mixture that will leave your hair shiny and healthy looking.

Chapter 7- Natural Beauty – Tips on Getting Rid of that Unwanted Gray Hair

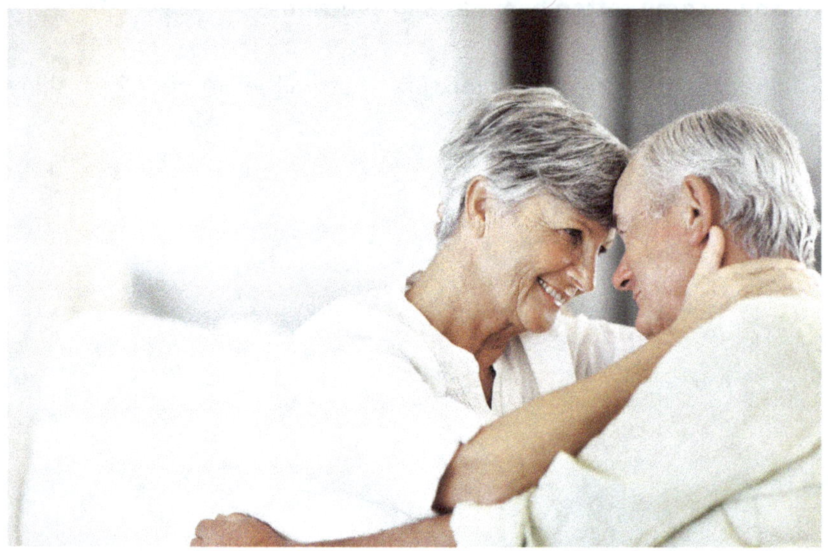

The first time you spot a gray hair, you may feel like you are aging before your time. Most people really start noticing their hair turning gray as they approach their late thirties. Some might be unlucky enough to experience gray hair much early. When you turn gray depends on the person and their genetics. However, there are things you can do to cover the gray.

Some people think that having gray hair makes them look more distinguished and do not wish to cover their new hair color. Most people are eager find ways to turn back the clock by using a variety of methods to cover the gray. If you are facing gray hair, consider the following tips for banishing the gray.

Hair turns gray as you age because your body experiences a natural slow-down of the production of pigment. Pigment in your hair gives you the color. As you age, this process slows and the natural color begins to fade. Not many people experience a full head of gray hair overnight. Instead, the process takes time, which results in gray hair mixed with color hair. Pulling out gray hair does not help. Instead, only another gray hair grows back to replace the pulled hair. Gray hair can also be less manageable because it becomes thicker, and coarser.

Gray hair also has decreased amounts of melanin, which naturally contains zinc, and iron that allows normal hair color to hold a dye. Therefore, gray hair can sometimes be harder to color. There are several steps you can take to help gray hair hold a hair color dye better and longer. Before coloring your gray hair you might want to take a minute to think about after care and maintenance. It is not always cheap or easy to continually color gray hair. If you do not want to make the commitment to color your hair every few weeks, then you should probably not dye your hair. You might even want to consider using color wands, which is similar to mascara. The color is not permanent but makes it easy and risk free to color gray strands.

Choose Your Dye Wisely

One common tip that helps cover gray hair is to choose a hair dye that is specifically made for gray hair. If your hair is not completely gray, then you will have a mixture of softer hair that is your natural color and the coarser gray hair. There are many styling products and hair dyes that are designed just for gray hair. This will help you have a better outcome, especially when you dye your hair at home.

Leave the Product in Longer

Leaving a hair dye in for just a little longer can help the hair retain the dye, resulting in a longer lasting dye job. It will be important to thoroughly read all of the instructions on the bottle. Most hair colors give specific instructions for dying gray hair and generally recommend leaving the dye on for at least 45 minutes. This will help all of the hair to be completely covered.

Pre-treat or Pre-soften the Hair

Gray hair is often resistant to color and a dye job may not last more than a few days. You can apply a 20% peroxide to help open the hair cuticles. This will allow the hair to soften and more readily accept the hair dye. It is a good idea to leave the peroxide on the hair for about 10 minutes, depending on the length of the hair in order for it to completely coat the hair.

Purchase Good Products

After you have successful colored your gray hair, shop for shampoos, conditioners and styling products that are specifically for gray hair or colored hair. Many stores, salons and boutiques carry these types of products. Using these maintenance products will help make a color last longer on stubborn gray hair.

Leave it to the professional: If the idea of using products and dyes at home scares you, leave it to the hair professional. There are many beauticians and salons that specialize in covering stubborn gray hair. Before you make an appointment, consider how much you want to spend and what color you want your hair. Have some ideas before your appointment and talk with your beautician to get ideas. You will get good results and usually a guarantee if you go with a professional.

Dye Jobs Gone Bad

Everyone can benefit from a great head of hair, whether it is a stylish new haircut or a great dye job. Great hair can boost self-esteem and make you feel like a million bucks. But what happens when you get an awful haircut or your dye job goes horribly wrong? Self-esteem hits rock bottom. Besides wearing a hat for the next three months, consider the following tips to ensure a healthy, attractive head of hair.

If you leave the hair salon or barbershop only to get home to notice an awful haircut, there are steps you can take to help you look your best. You probably will not be able to get your back, but you can return to the place or person who cut your hair and ask them for help. It might help to request a new beautician or to have the one that originally cut your hair show you ways to style your new hair-do. It could be that the haircut you got was what you wanted and you are just not styling it properly.

For hair that is cut too short, you may have to look at accessories to help style your hair while it is growing out. Small alligator clips are fashionable and can keep layers out of your face during the growing out period. In addition, if you get a haircut that is so short or so embarrassing, consider looking at synthetic hairpieces. Many stores carry clips, ponytails and other accessories with synthetic hair attached. They come in virtually every shade to match any color of hair.

Bad dye jobs can often be easier to fix than bad haircuts. If you are the recipient of an especially bad dye job there are a few steps you can take to correct the problem. First, if you have dyed your hair by yourself and find that you have under colored you hair, you probably rinsed too early. You can easily correct this problem by applying another dye to your hair and leave it in for the required time.

Over coloring your hair can be harder to correct. When this happens, it usually means that you have selected the wrong color for your hair or you have left the chemicals in too long. There are several products you can purchase that will help you take the color out of bad dye jobs. However, these products can be tricky to use and if you are afraid of the results, you might need to consult a professional. A beautician that specializes in hair color can help you correct your hair color without damaging the hair.

Another common hair problem does not have to do with bad haircuts or dye jobs, but with colored or blonde hair turning green when exposed to chlorine. This can be quite problematic, especially in the summer months. One way to correct this problem is to wash and shampoo hair right after swimming in chlorinated water. You can also help remove the green tint by purchasing a special product available through most retail and drug stores. If your hair is dyed or permed and it turns green, you may not be able to correct the problem at home. Seek the advice of a hair care professional before attempting to correct the problem at home.

There are preventative steps you can take to ensure you always have an attractive head of hair. If you are ready to change hairstyles, on tip is to make sure you understand what styles work best for your face shape. Also, consider using a beautician you know and can trust. Never have a drastic hair cut or dyed by someone you have never seen before. Also, have pictures available of what you expect your hair to look like, but at the same time, have realistic expectations. Not everyone can have the hairstyle of a movie star and expect to look that good. You will need to learn how to style the new cut and how to take care of the color.

Another good tip is to use products that are appropriate for your hair. If you have dyed blonde hair, look for shampoos and styling products specifically for dyed blonde hair. These types of products can help you keep the color longer. The right styling products are a must for certain hairstyles, too. Ask your hair care professional what is right for your new haircut.

Chapter 8 Natural Beauty – Treating that Dandruff Naturally

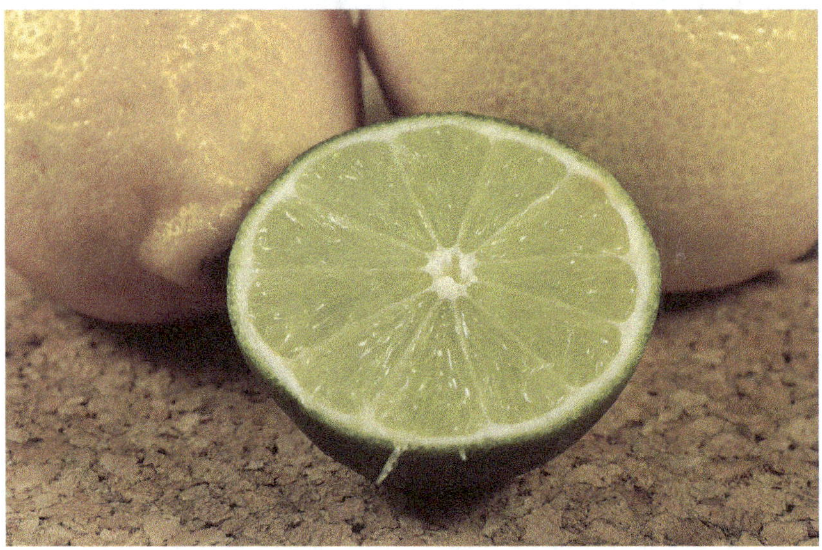

Dandruff is a skin condition where shiny, silvery, scales separate from the scalp and collect in the hair and fall into your brows, shoulders, and clothes. This condition becomes a problem when skin gets infected. The best remedy is to keep the hair and scalp clean to keep dead cells from accumulating. Getting a bit of sunshine may also aid in keeping dandruff at bay.

Dandruff Symptoms

The scales from the scalp fall when the hair is combed or brushed, or when the scalp is scratched, the scales from the scalp fall like snowflakes and settle on the eye brows, shoulders, and clothes. These scales sometimes appear as lumps or crusts on the scalp.

Itching is there and scalp may become red.

Often there is itching as well and the scalp may become red from scratching.

Dandruff Causes

Impairment of general health, wrong food intake, constipation.

The main causes of dandruff are impairment of general health, development of a toxic condition mainly due to taking of wrong foods, constipation, and a low vitality due to infectious diseases.

Emotional Tension, Harsh Shampoos, General Exhaustion

Other factors contributing to this disorder are emotional tension, harsh shampoos, exposure to cold and general exhaustion.

Home Remedies for Dandruff

Dandruff treatment using Fenugreek Seeds

The use of fenugreek seeds is one of the most important remedies in the treatment of dandruff. Two tablespoons of these seeds should be soaked overnight in water and ground into a fine paste in the morning. This paste should be applied all over the scalp and left for half an hour. The hair should then be washed thoroughly with soap-nut (ritha) solution or shikakai.

Dandruff Treatment using Lime

The use of a teaspoon of fresh lime juice for the last rinse, while washing the hair, is another useful remedy. This not only leaves the hair glowing but also removes stickiness and prevents dandruff.

Dandruff Treatment using Green Gram Powder

A valuable prescription for removal of dandruff is the use of green gram powder. The hair should be washed twice a week with two tablespoons of this powder mixed with half a cup of curd.

Dandruff Treatment using Beet

Beets have been found useful in dandruff. Both tops and roots should be boiled in water and this water should be massaged into the scalp with the finger tips every night. White beet is better for this purpose.

Dandruff Treatment using Snake Gourd

The juice of snake gourd has been found beneficial in the prevention and treatment of dandruff. The juice should be rubbed over the scalp for this purpose.

Dandruff Treatment using Other Remedies

Dandruff can be removed by massaging the hair for half an hour with curd which has been kept in the open for three days, or with a few drops of lime juice mixed with lime juice every night, before going to bed. Another measure which helps to counteract dandruff is to dilute cider vinegar with an equal quantity of water and dab this on to the hair with cotton wool in between shampooing. Cider vinegar added to the final rinsing water after shampooing also helps to disperse dandruff.

Anti-Dandruff Diet

All-fruit diet with three meals a day of juicy fruits.

Diet plays an important role in the treatment of dandruff. To begin with, the patient should resort to an all-fruit diet for about five days and take three meals a day of juicy fruits.

Avoid citrus fruits, bananas, tinned fruits: Citrus fruits, bananas, dried, stewed, or tinned fruits should not be taken.

Well-balanced diet

After the all-fruit diet, the patient can gradually adopt a well-balanced diet, with emphasis on raw foods, especially fresh fruits and vegetables. Further short periods of an all-fruit diet for three days or so may be necessary at monthly intervals till the skin's condition improves.

Avoid strong tea/coffee, pickles, refined and processed foods.

Meats, sugar, white flour, strong tea or coffee, condiments, pickles, refined and processed foods should all be avoided.

Other Dandruff treatments

Keep hair and scalp clean to avoid accumulation of dead cells.

The foremost consideration in the treatment of this disorder is to keep the hair and scalp clean so as to minimize the accumulation of dead cells.

Hair should be brushed daily to improve circulation

The hair should be brushed daily to improve the circulation and remove any flakiness. The most effective way to brush the hair is to bend forward from the waist with the head down towards the ground, and brush from the nape of the neck towards the top of the head. The scalp should also be thoroughly massaged everyday, using one's finger tips and working systematically over the head. This should be done just before or after brushing the hair. Like brushing, this stimulates the circulation, dislodges dirt and dandruff, and encourages hair growth. Exposure of the head to the rays of the sun is also a useful measure in the treatment of dandruff.

CHAPTER 9- NATURAL BEAUTY – DEALING WITH YOUR EYES, LIPS AND BROWS

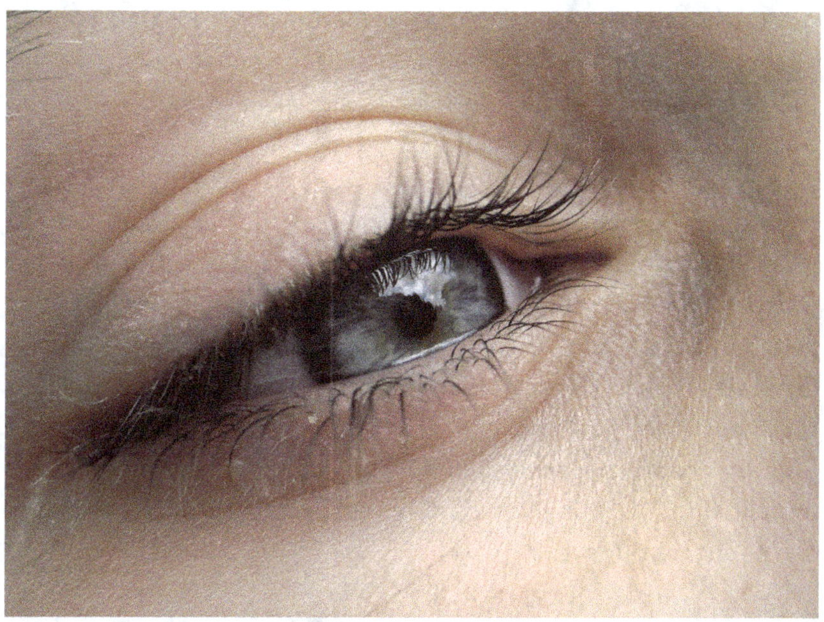

The dreaded look in the mirror shows the dark circles under your eyes. What are you supposed to do about it? If you have to look great, there may be a few ways that you can greatly improve these dark circles under your eyes. What causes them to happen? Sometimes this is hereditary, and there is very little you can do about those dark circles. They can also be caused by a lack of sleep or not getting enough water. Dehydration is one of the key and most common reasons for dark circles under the eyes.

Naturally Get Rid Of Them

Of course, the most important way to get rid of dark circles is to get more sleep and to drink more water. This process can take some time, though. You'll need a few hours of sleep and you should try to drive up to eight glasses of water each day. Look for all natural skin care products, too. These can give you a lot of help in hiding the dark circles when you are unable to otherwise improve them. A good place to start is with a natural moisturizer. This aids in providing more moisture to the skin in this area which can cause the dark circles to fad. Look for products that contain Vitamin K, sesame oil, Vitamin E and avocado oil. These are a great choice to use on a regular basis, too, especially under your make up if you are prone to dark circles.

A variety of concealers are on the market that will work well to mask the dark circles under your eyes. Take a good look at the product. Choose something that is actually all natural, if it is possible to do so. Do make sure to choose the right color concealer. If you do not, you could risk making the dark circles stand out more so. Choose a natural color that matches your skin well. Or, choose a concealer that is just one shade lighter than your foundation. This will give you the best results in hiding the dark circles under your eyes.

When it comes to hiding your dark circles, keep in mind that there are many ways to do so, but the best way is to take steps to help you to stop them from happening. In other words, get some sleep and drink water, too. Your beautiful skin does not need to be marred by dark circles.

Chapped Lips? How To Avoid This Problem

Chapped lips are one of the first signs of the winter months and they can be one of the most difficult health problems to overcome. When your lips are chapped, you want to wet them over and over again since this action actually seems to sooth them. The problem is, as they dry, the wetting them has made them worse. What can you do to overcome this? In addition, what options are there for avoiding dry lips in the first place?

Treating Chapped Lips

As a fashion statement or a beauty statement, there is o doubt that chapped lips are a big no-no. The pealing and the pain they cause are going to make any lipstick that you apply over them hard to remove and horrible to look at. You may even get a burning sensation if you tried to cover them up. The best way to treat them is with a soothing, medicated chap stick or lip balm. These are found at most location where medications are sold. Avoid products that are sugar based or that are made for children. What ou are looking for is a specific, medicated product that will place a very small dose of medication into these wounds to help them heal. They also work to lock in the moisture on your lips. Apply as often as needed until the painful cracks have healed.

Avoiding It

The only thing better than improving chapped lips is to actually be able to avoid getting them. In many cases, you can do this. First, be sure you stay hydrated. If your body is not hydrated the skin, and the lip, cells will become dry, leaving them highly vulnerable to wind and cold weather. Second, cover up. When heading outdoors in the cold weather, wear a scarf around your face. This is especially true of very low temperatures, also when the wind is blowing.

Next, apply a layer of moisture protection to your lips. Choose a lip balm, not necessarily one that is medicated, to keep your lips moist. These products are important because of the close proximity to your mouth (the moisture there is what ends up causing the chapped feeling.)

Stop licking your lips. Avoid having this big beauty problem. Simply treat your lips with these products so that you can use lipsticks again. You should avoid these products if you have chapped lips since they can worsen the situation.

How To Have Great Eyebrows

You may not notice them often but your eyebrows really do make a statement about you. They show off your eyes and help to accentuate your overall looks. When you take the time to have great looking eyebrows, the end result is a face that is well made and well groomed. It does not have to be difficult to have great looking eyebrows like this, either.

When should you pluck your eyebrows? Does it matter? In fact it does matter. Eyebrows that are plucked should be plucked right before you go to bed. This allows for the redness caused by the plucking to fade overnight. In the morning, you will have great looking eyebrows without any swelling or redness.

Here are some more tips and hints to having great looking eyebrows:

• If you have never done your eyebrows yourself, talk with your beautician first. Not only will they do it for you, but they can help teach you how to do it. This way, you know how to shape them and how to pluck them.

• Be sure to use the right tools for the process. Purchase a pair of slant edge tweezers to aid you.

These work well because they can easily grab your hair. Plus, you will need a small comb. Prior to doing any plucking, comb all of the eyebrow hair in one direction. This helps to separate them so that you can easily remove them.

• Clean up after you have finished. You will need to look just outside the normal row of hairs for your eyebrows. There may be stray pieces hiding to remove. Also, in between your two eyebrows needs to be cleaned up. Pluck any stray hairs in this region.

• Don't overdo it. You can over pluck your eyebrows. This especially is possible if you haven't taken the steps to play which hairs to pluck and have just kept working to try and even the brows out. Instead, use an eye pencil first to draw out where you want to trim and remove. This way, you are less likely to over pluck.

Taking care of your eyebrows does not need to be difficult. In fact, if you just invest a few minutes after or before you wash your face each night, chances are good you will have a great look regularly. Eyebrows, often forgotten, but they do not have to be

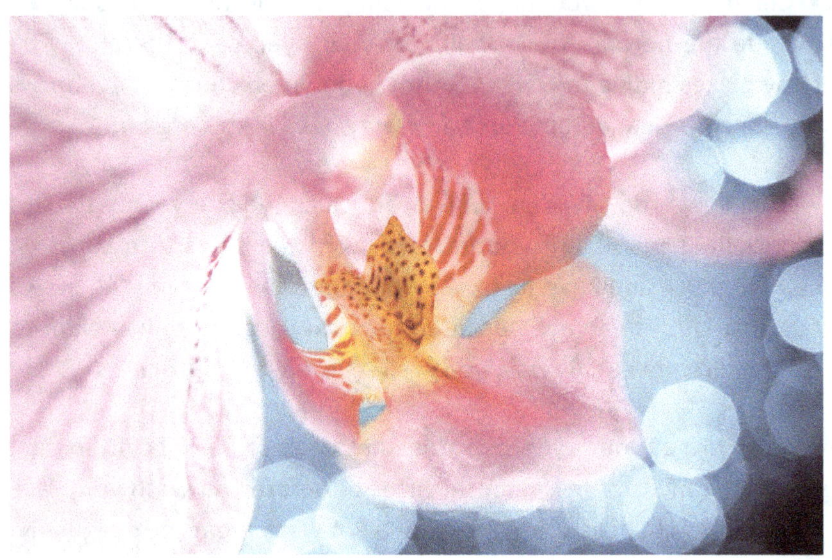

1. Apple Tart Soap

4oz. Clear, Unscented Glycerine Soap

1 Tablespoon Liquid Soap

1 teaspoon Liquid Glycerine

1/2 teaspoon Apple Fragrance Oil

2 Drops Red Food Color

1/2 teaspoon Ground Cinnamon

Melt soap in small pan over low heat or in a glass cup in the microwave.

Add Liquid Soap and glycerin and stir gently but well. Add fragrance, color and cinnamon. Stir and let stand a couple minutes, just enough to start to thicken so when you stir again the cinnamon will be more evenly distributed.

Pour into molds. Allow to set completely (in or out of freezer).

Wrap in plastic wrap or use cellophane candy bags.

2. Apricot Freesia Tarts

Ingredients For Tart:

1 lb White Glycerin Soap Base

12 Drops Cosmic Color Canary Yellow

11 Drops Cosmic Color Red

1 t. Apricot Freesia FO

Ingredients For "Whipped Cream" Topping:

4 oz White Glycerin Soap Base

¼ t. Apricot Freesia FO

A "Shake" of Super Sparkle Gold Sparkle DustTM

Melt soap base for tart in a double boiler.

Once melted, add color and fragrance.

Pour into a muffin tin and allow to harden.

Remove from tin.Melt soap base for topping and add a shake of Sparkle

Dust.

With an electric mixer, mix until thick and bubbly.

Spray tarts with rubbing alcohol and spoon the topping onto the tarts while allowing some to run over tarts.

Top with a dash of Sparkle Dust if desired.

3. Aspen Dreams Bath Salts

This scent is very woody, and is suited for soothing your muscles and relaxing in the tub. It is very masculine in scent, I think. I enjoy this after a long day at work; it makes me feel comfortable and content. Women love it as well as men do.

The ingredients are:

2 cups of Epsom salts (or a mixture epsom/sea)

2 tablespoons of baking soda

essential oils:

5 drops of rosewood

2 drops cedarwood

2 drops Chamomile

a nice jar with a tight fitting lid

To make the salts:

Mix the salts and baking soda in a bowl very well.

Mix oils in a small cup. Take them and pour them evenly over the salt.

Mix the two very well.

Let sit for over an hour before placing in a jar and sealing.

If you are going to color these use yellow and red to make a light brown.

4. Balancing Bath Salts

Sea Salt--3 tbsp

Baking Soda--3 tbsp

Essential Oils--8 drops

Jar--4 oz

Choose 3 or 4 oils from these essential oils: Bergamot, Frankincense,

Geranium, Lavender, Palmarosa, Rose, and Rosewood.

Add sea salt, baking soda and oils to jar. Gently shake to mix, mix well.

Add to tub of running water.

5. Balancing Epson Salt Bath

Epson Salt--2 tbsp

Sea Salt--1 tbsp

Baking Soda--3 tbsp

Essential Oils--8 drops

Jar--4 oz

Choose 3 or 4 oils from these essential oils: Bergamot, Frankincense,

Geranium, Lavender, Palmarosa, Rose, and Rosewood.

Add sea salt, baking soda, epson salts and oils to jar. Gently shake to mix, mix well. Add to tub of running water.

6. Balancing Fizzy Bath Salts

Sea Salt--3 tbsp

Baking Soda--3 tbsp

Citric Acid--1 tbsp

Essential Oils--8 drops

Jar--4 oz

Choose 3 or 4 oils from these essential oils: Bergamot, Frankincense,

Geranium, Lavender, Palmarosa, Rose, and Rosewood.

Add sea salt, baking soda, citric acid and oils to jar. Gently shake to mix, mix well. Add to tub of running water.

7. Balancing Red Earth Salts

Sea Salt--2 tbsp

Baking Soda--3 tbsp

Powdered Red Earth Clay--1 tbsp

Essential Oils--8 drops

Jar--4 oz

Choose 3 or 4 oils from these essential oils: Bergamot, Frankincense,

Geranium, Lavender, Palmarosa, Rose, and Rosewood.

Add sea salt, baking soda, powdered red earth clay and oils to jar. Gently shake to mix, mix well. Add to tub of running water.

8. Balancing Seaweed Salts

Sea Salt--2 tbsp

Baking Soda--3 tbsp

Powdered Kelp--1 tbsp

Essential Oils--8 drops

Jar--4 oz

Choose 3 or 4 oils from these essential oils: Bergamot, Frankincense,

Geranium, Lavender, Palmarosa, Rose, and Rosewood.

Add sea salt, baking soda, powdered kelp and oils to jar. Gently shake to mix, mix well. Add to tub of running water.

9. Basic Bubble Bath

Ingredients:

5 drops fragrant oil or essential oil (your choice)

1 quart water

1 bar castille soap (grated or flaked)

1 1/2 ounces glycerin

Directions:

Mix all ingredients together. Store in a container. Pour in running water.

10. Basil and Lime Bath Salts

You will need:

5 cups of Sea Salt (or Epsom salt, or a combination of both)

1 Tsp. of Baking Powder

2 Tsp. of Almond Oil

5 drops Lime Scented Oil

4 drops Basil Oil

1 drop green coloring

1 drop yellow coloring

All you have to do is mix the salt and the baking powder in a bowl. In another smaller bowl mix together all liquids and add to salts, stirring well. You should let them sit so they can soak up the scent and the coloring allof the way through. After they have sat for about two hours take them and placethem in jars with cork stoppers. To create a good seal dip the cork in melted wax (greento match salts) and put cork into bottle.

11. Bath Cookies

2 cups finely ground sea salt

1/2 cup baking soda

1/2 cup cornstarch

2 tbs. light oil

1 tsp. vitamin E oil

2 eggs

5-6 drops essential oil

Preheat oven to 350 F. Mix together all the ingredients. Take a teaspoon of the dough and roll it gently into a ball about 1" in diameter. Continue doing this with all the dough and place the balls on an ungreased cookie sheet. (You can decorate the cookies with clove buds, anise seeds, or dried citurs peel if you wish.) Bake the cookies for 10 minutes, until they are lightly browned. Do not overbake. Allow the cookies to cool completely.

To use, drop 1 or 2 cookies into a warm bath and allow to dissolve. Do not eat! Yield: 24 cookies, enough for 12+ baths.

12. Bath Bombs / Bath Fizzies

2 tbs. citric acid (you can get this at a pharmacy)

2 tbs. cornstarch

1/4 cup baking soda

3 tbs. coconut oil (or any other emollient oil like almond, avocado or apricot kernel oil)

1/4 tsp. fragrance oil

3-6 drops of food coloring (if desired)

Paper candy cups

Place all of the dry ingredients (first 3) into a bowl and mix well. Place coconut oil into a small glass bowl and add fragrance and food coloring.

Slowly add oil mixture into dry ingredients and mix well. Scoop up small amounts of the mixture and shape into 1" balls. Let the balls rest on a sheet of waxed paper for about 2 to 3 hours, then place each ball into a candy cup to let dry and harden for 24 to 48 hours. Store bombs in a closed, air-tight container. To use, drop 1 to 3 bombs into warm bath water.

13. Bridal Bath Salts

(in 4 layers ~ makes 16oz.)

2 Cups Rock Salt

1/2 Teaspoon of Each Fragrance Oil

Rose, Sage, Lavender, Rosemary

Food Color

Divide salt into four equal amounts, place each in a container with sealable lids. That's 1/2 cup in each container or for 8 ounces of bath salts use ¼ cup in each container and half the amount of fragrance oil and food color.

Add 1/2 teaspoon Rose fragrance oil and 4 Drops of red food color (or you can leave it white), put lid on and shake well. To the next one add 1/2teaspoon Chamomile-Sage (or just sage if you have it) and 4 drops of green and 2 drops of blue food color and shake. To the third add 1/2 teaspoon Lavender fragrance oil, 3 drops of red and 4 drops of blue food color and shake well. To the last container add ½ teaspoon Rosemary fragrance oil, 4-8 drops of green food color and shake. On separate pieces of wax paper, spread out each color and air dry for several hours. When the salt is completely dry layer it in the container. Rosemary ~ Lavender ~ Sage ~ Rose (on top) To speed up the drying process you can put the wax paper on a cookie sheet and put it in the oven and let the pilot light work on it or for an electric oven, pre-heat at lowest temperature and turn off before putting salt in the oven. You have just made lovely layered bath salts that also has special meaning. Red Rose - Means Unity White Rose - Represents Pure Spiritual Love Sage - Represents Good Health and Long Life Lavender - Means Devotion

Rosemary - Lasting Friendship and Remembrance

14. Bubble Bags

Used in the shower, when there is no time to take a soaking bath.

2 parts oatmeal

2 parts dried herbs

1 part grated soap

Place ingredients in a cloth bag and use as a washcloth

15. Candy Cane Bath Salts

Ingredients:

3 cups of Epsom salts

3 Teaspoons of Sweet Almond Oil

9 drops of Peppermint Essential Oil

1 drop of red food coloring (more if you like)

1 drop of green food coloring

To decorate:

several jars with turn lids or cork seals

red, green and white Christmas ribbon

several gift tags shaped like candy canes OR

several candy canes (small ones)

To make the salts separate each of the three cups of salts into three bowls.

Separate each teaspoon of almond oil into three bowls.

Into one bowl of almond oil add the drop of red food coloring; into the second add the green. Into each of the three bowls of oil add three drops of peppermint oil. Mix each bowl well. After mixing pour each of the bowls of oils and coloring into one of the bowls of salt. This will leave you with a bowl of green a bowl of red and a bowl of white scented salts. Let sit for a few hours covered.

To create the candy cane effect layer layers of each color, a layer of red, a layer of green , a layer of white, over and over until you fill the jar.

16. Candy Cane Swirl

You will need:

½ lb. MP opaque base

1 tsp. Stearic acid

red colorant

Candy Cane fragrance oil

candy cane cookie cutters

wax paper lined pan or tray

**you could also use the Wilton mini cake pan candy cane mold

Melt the MP base and stearic acid separately. Combine them when they are

both liquefied. Whisk well. Add the fragrance oil and pour into a wax paper lined pan or tray. Take a bit of red coloring (just a bit on the tip of the toothpick) and swirl into the soap until it is marblized. When it is firm enough, take cookie cutter and cut out candy cane shapes. These are great for Christmas!!!

17. Chamomile Fields Shampoo

4 bags of chamomile tea (or 1 handful of fresh chamomile flowers)

4 tbs. pure soap flakes

1-1/2 tbs. glycerin

Let the tea bags steep in 1-1/2 cups boiled water for 10 minutes. Remove the tea bags and with the remaining liquid add the soap flakes. Let stand until the soap softens. Stir in glycerin until mixture is well blended.

Pour into a bottle. Keep in a dark, cool place.

18. Champagne Bubble Bath

1/4 C foaming concentrate

3/4 C distilled water

1/2 tsp. table salt(not sea salt)

1 TBSP. glycerin

1/4 tsp. Champagne or white wine fragrance oil

Buy a split of champagne- drink it or toss it but keep the bottle. Heat water(not boiling just hot), stir in concentrate and glycerin until completely dissolved. Add fragrance oil and stir well. Add salt stirring until dissolved. Allow mixture to cool. If itis not as thick as you would like add another 1/4 tsp. salt stirring until dissolved pour into a clean champagne split and seal bottle. Using a pink or white paint pen create labels for the front and back on gold stickers. with a square of candy foil cover the cork, twisting at the neck

19. Camphor and Clary Sage Soap

2 c. M&P soap base

2 T. camphor oil

1/4 c. clary sage infusion

AND/OR

1 tsp. clary sage oil

Combine melted soap and herbal ingredients. Stir until blended, and pour into molds. Keep soap wrapped or store in a cool dark place. It will be good for about 18 months. Note: This also works well for poison Ivy.

20. Cherry Berry Bubble Bath

1/2 cup unscented shampoo

3/4 cup water

1/2 tsp. salt (regular table salt is fine)

15 drops cherry fragrance oil

Pour shampoo into a bowl and add water. Stir gently until well mixed. Add salt, and stir until mixture thickens. Add cherry fragrance oil and place in decorative bottle. Can also be used as a body wash!

ABOUT THE AUTHOR

Susan Johnson is a mother of three. She has two lovely daughters and a good looking son. Susan is a natural beauty expert. She believes that there is always a natural way on how to take care of oneself without having to rely on chemical based beauty products. At a very young age, she started making her own beauty recipes.

Currently Susan is cooking another beauty regimen book together with her eldest daughter. Writing these kinds of books to share to others is something that Susan really loves. She wants to be an instrument to all that beauty doesn't need to be painful and expensive.

www.ingramcontent.com/pod-product-compliance
Lightning Source LLC
Chambersburg PA
CBHW070042260726
48658CB00002B/695